The Glucose Goddess Method

A Comprehensive Guide to Regulate
Your Blood Sugar Levels, Transform Your
Health and Regain Stamina

Margaret R. Harris

Table of Contents

Introduction

Welcome to "The Glucose Goddess Method: A Comprehensive Guide to Regulate Your Blood Sugar Levels, Transform Your Health, and Regain Stamina." In this book, we will embark on a journey to understand the vital role that blood sugar regulation plays in achieving optimal health and vitality.

Maintaining balanced blood sugar levels is a cornerstone of overall well-being, as it influences various aspects of our physical and mental health. However, in today's fast-paced world filled with processed foods, sedentary lifestyles, and increasing stress levels, many individuals struggle with blood sugar imbalances that can have far-reaching consequences.

"The Glucose Goddess Method" is designed to empower you with knowledge, practical strategies, and actionable steps to regain control over your blood sugar levels and transform your health. Whether you are already dealing with blood sugar-related issues or simply looking to prevent future problems, this comprehensive guide will provide you with the tools you need to make positive changes.

Throughout this book, we will explore the science behind blood sugar regulation, demystifying key concepts and providing you with a solid foundation of understanding. You will learn how factors like insulin, glycemic index, and dietary choices impact your blood sugar levels, and why it is crucial to maintain stability for long-term health.

"The Glucose Goddess Method" is rooted in four pillars of blood sugar balance: nutrition, exercise, stress management, and tracking. By addressing these fundamental aspects of your lifestyle, you will embark on a holistic approach to achieving and sustaining balanced blood sugar levels.

In each chapter, we will delve into practical strategies and expert guidance, enabling you to make informed choices and take proactive steps towards a healthier future. From optimizing your diet to incorporating exercise routines that support blood sugar regulation, and from managing stress effectively to tracking your progress, this book provides you with a comprehensive roadmap to success.

Remember, this journey is not about temporary fixes or restrictive measures. It is about adopting sustainable lifestyle changes that will become second nature to you. It is about reclaiming your health, revitalizing your energy, and regaining your stamina. With "The Glucose Goddess Method" as your guide, you will be equipped with the knowledge and tools necessary to achieve lasting wellness and become the best version of yourself.

So, let us embark on this transformative journey together, empowering you to regulate your blood sugar levels, transform your health, and embrace a vibrant, energetic life.

What is the Glucose Method?

The Glucose Goddess Method is a comprehensive approach to regulating blood sugar levels and achieving overall health and vitality. It is a system that combines scientific knowledge, practical strategies, and lifestyle changes to support balanced blood sugar and optimize well-being.

At its core, the Glucose Goddess Method recognizes the significant impact that blood sugar levels have on various aspects of our health. When our blood sugar is stable, we experience increased energy levels, improved mood, better cognitive function, and enhanced physical performance. On the other hand, imbalances in blood sugar can lead to a range of health issues, including weight gain, fatigue, mood swings, and an increased risk of chronic conditions such as diabetes and cardiovascular disease.

The Glucose Goddess Method emphasizes four pillars of blood sugar balance: nutrition, exercise, stress management, and tracking. By addressing these key areas, individuals can gain better control over their blood sugar levels and experience improved health outcomes.

1. Nutrition: The Glucose Goddess Method emphasizes the importance of a balanced and nutrient-rich diet. It encourages the consumption of whole, unprocessed foods that are low on the glycemic index, which helps to prevent spikes in blood sugar. The method also provides guidance on portion control, meal planning, and the incorporation of specific superfoods and

supplements that support blood sugar regulation.

2. Exercise: Physical activity plays a crucial role in blood sugar control. The Glucose Goddess Method emphasizes the importance of regular exercise, including both cardiovascular and strength training activities. Exercise helps to improve insulin sensitivity, allowing for better utilization of glucose by the body's cells and promoting stable blood sugar levels.

3. Stress Management: Chronic stress can disrupt blood sugar levels by triggering the release of stress hormones such as cortisol. The Glucose Goddess Method focuses on stress management techniques such as relaxation exercises, mindfulness practices, and adequate sleep. By reducing stress levels, individuals can support more stable blood sugar regulation.

4. Tracking: Monitoring and tracking blood sugar levels are vital components of the Glucose Goddess Method. By regularly measuring blood sugar levels and keeping a food and mood diary, individuals can gain valuable insights into the effects of their lifestyle choices on their blood sugar. This tracking helps to identify patterns, make necessary adjustments, and celebrate progress along the journey towards blood sugar balance.

By implementing the Glucose Goddess Method, individuals can take control of their blood sugar levels and experience transformative changes in their health and well-being. The method provides a holistic and sustainable approach, empowering individuals to make informed choices, adopt healthy habits, and ultimately reclaim their vitality.

Understanding the Importance of Blood Sugar Regulation

Blood sugar regulation is a fundamental process in the human body that plays a crucial role in maintaining overall health and well-being. It refers to the control and balance of glucose levels in the bloodstream, ensuring that they remain within a narrow range for optimal functioning.

Glucose, a type of sugar derived from the carbohydrates we consume, serves as the primary source of energy for our cells. It fuels our brain, muscles, and organs, providing the necessary energy for daily activities and bodily functions.

When blood sugar levels are properly regulated, several benefits emerge:

1. Stable Energy Levels: Balanced blood sugar levels provide a steady supply of glucose to the cells, ensuring a consistent

energy source throughout the day. This stability helps prevent energy crashes, fatigue, and mood swings that can occur when blood sugar levels fluctuate erratically.

2. Weight Management: Blood sugar regulation is closely linked to weight management. When blood sugar levels rise too high, insulin, a hormone produced by the pancreas, is released to facilitate the absorption of glucose into the cells. Insulin also signals the body to store excess glucose as fat. By maintaining stable blood sugar levels, the risk of overeating and weight gain can be minimized.

3. Cognitive Function: The brain heavily relies on glucose for optimal cognitive function. When blood sugar levels are balanced, the brain receives a consistent supply of glucose, supporting mental clarity, concentration, and memory. On the contrary, fluctuations in blood sugar can

impair cognitive performance and contribute to brain fog or difficulty focusing.

4. Disease Prevention: Proper blood sugar regulation plays a pivotal role in preventing and managing various health conditions. Chronic high blood sugar levels, such as those seen in diabetes, can lead to complications affecting the heart, blood vessels, kidneys, eyes, and nerves. By maintaining stable blood sugar levels, the risk of developing diabetes and its associated complications can be significantly reduced.

5. Mood Stability: Blood sugar imbalances can affect mood and emotional well-being. Sharp spikes and crashes in blood sugar levels can contribute to irritability, anxiety, and mood swings. Achieving stable blood sugar regulation can help promote a more balanced emotional state.

Understanding the importance of blood sugar regulation underscores the significance of adopting a proactive approach to achieve and maintain balance. By incorporating healthy lifestyle choices, such as consuming a balanced diet, engaging in regular physical activity, managing stress effectively, and monitoring blood sugar levels, individuals can take charge of their health and promote stable blood sugar regulation.

Chapter 1

The Science Behind Blood Sugar

Understanding the science behind blood sugar is essential for comprehending the mechanisms involved in its regulation and the impact it has on our overall health. Blood sugar, or blood glucose, refers to the concentration of glucose present in the bloodstream at any given time. Glucose is a sugar molecule that serves as the primary source of energy for the body's cells.

The Role of Insulin:
Insulin, a hormone produced by the pancreas, plays a central role in blood sugar regulation. When we consume carbohydrates, they are broken down into glucose during digestion. As glucose enters the bloodstream, the pancreas releases

insulin in response to rising blood sugar levels.

Insulin acts as a key that unlocks the cells, allowing glucose to enter and be utilized for energy production. It helps transport glucose from the bloodstream into cells, particularly in the muscles, liver, and adipose tissue. In these cells, glucose is either used immediately for energy or stored for later use.

Glycemic Index:
The glycemic index (GI) is a measure of how quickly carbohydrates in food raise blood sugar levels. Foods with a high GI value cause a rapid spike in blood sugar, while those with a low GI value result in a slower, more gradual increase. Consuming predominantly high-GI foods can lead to more significant fluctuations in blood sugar levels and may strain the body's insulin response over time.

Glucose Homeostasis:
The body maintains blood sugar levels within a narrow range to ensure proper functioning. This process, known as glucose homeostasis, involves a delicate balance of various hormones and mechanisms.

When blood sugar levels rise, such as after a meal, the pancreas releases insulin to facilitate the uptake of glucose into cells, thereby reducing blood sugar levels. In contrast, when blood sugar levels drop, the pancreas releases another hormone called glucagon, which triggers the release of stored glucose from the liver to elevate blood sugar levels.

Additionally, the liver plays a critical role in maintaining blood sugar balance. It acts as a storage site for glycogen, a complex carbohydrate formed by glucose molecules. When blood sugar levels decrease, the liver breaks down glycogen into glucose and releases it into the bloodstream, helping to prevent hypoglycemia.

The Impact of Blood Sugar Imbalances: When blood sugar regulation is disrupted, it can have significant implications for health. Chronic high blood sugar levels, as seen in conditions like diabetes, can lead to various complications, including cardiovascular disease, kidney damage, nerve damage, and eye problems. On the other hand, frequent episodes of low blood sugar (hypoglycemia) can cause dizziness, confusion, and, in severe cases, loss of consciousness.

Maintaining Blood Sugar Balance: Achieving and maintaining blood sugar balance is crucial for overall health and well-being. It involves making conscious dietary choices, including consuming a balanced diet rich in whole grains, lean proteins, healthy fats, and plenty of fruits and vegetables. Engaging in regular physical activity, managing stress levels, and getting adequate sleep also contribute to blood sugar regulation.

Demystifying Blood Sugar: What You Need to Know

Blood sugar, also known as blood glucose, is a vital component of our body's functioning, playing a crucial role in energy production and overall health. Understanding the basics of blood sugar is essential for maintaining optimal well-being and preventing imbalances that can lead to various health complications. Let's demystify blood sugar and explore what you need to know.

1. What is Blood Sugar?
Blood sugar refers to the concentration of glucose, a type of sugar, in the bloodstream. Glucose serves as the primary source of energy for our cells and is derived from the

carbohydrates we consume in our diet. After digestion, glucose is absorbed into the bloodstream, where it circulates to reach different cells and organs.

2. Why is Blood Sugar Regulation Important?

Proper blood sugar regulation is vital because glucose needs to be available in the bloodstream at appropriate levels to fuel the body's functions. Too much or too little glucose in the bloodstream can disrupt normal bodily processes and have negative consequences for our health.

3. Insulin and Blood Sugar Control:

Insulin, a hormone produced by the pancreas, plays a central role in blood sugar control. When blood sugar levels rise after a meal, the pancreas releases insulin into the bloodstream. Insulin helps glucose enter the cells, where it can be used for energy or stored for later use. This process lowers blood sugar levels and maintains stability.

4. Glycemic Index (GI):
The glycemic index (GI) is a scale that measures how quickly carbohydrates in foods raise blood sugar levels. Foods with a high GI value cause a more rapid and significant increase in blood sugar, while low GI foods lead to a slower and more gradual rise. Choosing low GI foods can help maintain stable blood sugar levels and provide sustained energy.

5. Blood Sugar Imbalances and Health Effects:
Both high and low blood sugar levels can have adverse effects on health. Chronic high blood sugar levels, as seen in diabetes, can lead to complications such as cardiovascular disease, nerve damage, kidney problems, and eye conditions. Low blood sugar levels (hypoglycemia) can cause symptoms like weakness, confusion, dizziness, and in severe cases, loss of consciousness.

6. Monitoring and Managing Blood Sugar: Monitoring blood sugar levels is important for individuals with diabetes or those aiming to maintain optimal health. Regular monitoring allows for early detection of imbalances, facilitating appropriate lifestyle adjustments and medical interventions when necessary. Lifestyle factors such as a balanced diet, regular exercise, stress management, and adequate sleep can all contribute to stable blood sugar levels.

By understanding the basics of blood sugar, its regulation, and the impact of imbalances, individuals can make informed choices about their lifestyle and dietary habits to promote optimal blood sugar control.

Insulin's Function in Blood Sugar Regulation

Insulin, a hormone produced by the pancreas, plays a critical role in regulating blood sugar levels in the body. It acts as a key player in the complex process of maintaining glucose homeostasis, ensuring that blood sugar remains within a narrow range for optimal health and functioning. Let's explore the role of insulin in blood sugar regulation.

1. Glucose Uptake: When we consume carbohydrates, they are broken down into glucose during digestion. After that, glucose is taken into the circulation, raising blood sugar levels. Insulin is then released into the bloodstream by the pancreas in response.

2. Cellular Uptake: Insulin acts as a key that unlocks the cells, allowing glucose to enter and be utilized for energy production. It facilitates the transport of glucose from the bloodstream into various cells of the body, including muscle, liver, and adipose (fat) tissue.

3. Muscle and Liver Storage: In muscle cells, insulin stimulates the uptake of glucose, where it can be converted into glycogen—a stored form of glucose. This glycogen can be broken down later to provide a readily available energy source during periods of increased energy demand, such as exercise. In the liver, insulin promotes the storage of excess glucose as glycogen as well.

4. Inhibition of Gluconeogenesis: Insulin also inhibits gluconeogenesis, which is the production of new glucose by the liver. By suppressing this process, insulin helps prevent excessive glucose production and release into the bloodstream, contributing to blood sugar stability.

5. Suppressing Glucagon Release: Insulin counteracts the action of another pancreatic hormone called glucagon. Blood sugar levels increase as a result of glucagon's stimulation of the liver to release glucose that has been

stored there. Insulin helps suppress the release of glucagon, preventing unnecessary increases in blood sugar.

6. Feedback Mechanism: The release of insulin is tightly regulated through a feedback mechanism. When blood sugar levels are high, such as after a meal, the pancreas secretes insulin to lower blood sugar. As blood sugar levels decrease, insulin secretion decreases accordingly, preventing blood sugar from dropping too low.

7. Insulin Resistance and Diabetes: In some cases, the body's cells become less responsive to the effects of insulin, leading to a condition called insulin resistance. This condition impairs glucose uptake, resulting in elevated blood sugar levels. Insulin resistance is a hallmark of type 2 diabetes, a chronic metabolic disorder. In type 1 diabetes, the pancreas fails to produce

insulin, leading to a reliance on exogenous insulin injections.

Understanding the crucial role of insulin in blood sugar regulation highlights its significance in maintaining optimal health. By promoting glucose uptake, storage, and suppressing processes that increase blood sugar, insulin ensures a balance between energy supply and demand.

The Effect of the Glycemic Index on Blood Sugar Levels

The glycemic index (GI) is a valuable tool that measures the effect of carbohydrates in food on blood sugar levels. It provides insight into how quickly and significantly different foods can cause blood sugar to rise after consumption. Understanding the glycemic index and its impact on blood sugar levels can help individuals make informed dietary choices for better blood sugar control and overall health.

1. What is the Glycemic Index (GI)?
The glycemic index is a numerical scale that ranks carbohydrates based on their potential to raise blood sugar levels. Foods with a high GI value (over 70) digest quickly, which causes blood sugar levels to rise quickly. Foods with a low GI value (below 55) are digested more slowly, resulting in a more gradual and controlled rise in blood sugar.

2. The Impact of High-GI Foods:
Consuming high-GI foods causes a rapid spike in blood sugar levels, leading to a corresponding increase in insulin release from the pancreas. This sudden surge of insulin aims to facilitate the transport of glucose from the bloodstream into cells for energy utilization. However, this rapid rise in blood sugar followed by a surge of insulin can result in a subsequent drop in blood

sugar levels, leading to feelings of fatigue, hunger, and cravings. Moreover, repeated consumption of high-GI foods can contribute to insulin resistance and an increased risk of type 2 diabetes.

3. The Benefits of Low-GI Foods:
Low-GI foods are digested more slowly, causing a gradual and steady rise in blood sugar levels. This slower release of glucose into the bloodstream allows for better blood sugar control and sustained energy levels. Low-GI foods also promote a feeling of fullness and satiety, which can aid in weight management and prevent overeating. Additionally, incorporating more low-GI foods in the diet has been associated with a reduced risk of chronic diseases such as type 2 diabetes, cardiovascular disease, and certain types of cancer.

4. Factors Influencing Glycemic Index:
Several factors influence the glycemic index of a food, including its carbohydrate type,

structure, processing, and cooking method. Foods with complex carbohydrates, such as whole grains, legumes, and non-starchy vegetables, generally have a lower GI compared to foods with simple carbohydrates, like refined grains and sugary snacks. Processing methods that break down the structure of carbohydrates, such as milling or grinding, can increase the glycemic index. Cooking methods that soften carbohydrates, such as boiling or steaming, can lower the GI compared to foods consumed raw.

5. Glycemic Load:
In addition to the glycemic index, the concept of glycemic load (GL) takes into account the quantity of carbohydrates consumed. The glycemic load considers both the quality (GI) and quantity of carbohydrates in a specific serving of food. It provides a more accurate representation of the overall impact on blood sugar levels than the glycemic index alone.

Understanding the glycemic index and glycemic load can guide individuals in making healthier food choices. A diet rich in low-GI foods, such as whole grains, fruits, vegetables, and lean proteins, can help maintain stable blood sugar levels, promote satiety, and support overall health.

Chapter 2

Assessing Your Blood Sugar Levels

Monitoring and assessing your blood sugar levels is an essential practice for maintaining optimal health, particularly if you have a condition like diabetes or want to ensure stable blood sugar control. Regular assessment allows you to understand how your body responds to different factors and make informed decisions about lifestyle and dietary choices. Here are key considerations for assessing your blood sugar levels:

1. Self-Monitoring of Blood Glucose (SMBG):
Self-monitoring of blood glucose involves using a blood glucose meter to measure your blood sugar levels at home. This method typically requires pricking your finger to obtain a small blood sample and using test

strips to measure the glucose concentration. SMBG allows you to check your blood sugar levels at different times throughout the day, before or after meals, or as recommended by your healthcare provider.

2. Continuous Glucose Monitoring (CGM): Continuous glucose monitoring involves wearing a small device that continuously measures your blood sugar levels throughout the day and night. It provides real-time data, offering a more comprehensive understanding of your blood sugar patterns and trends. CGM systems use a tiny sensor inserted under the skin to measure glucose levels in the interstitial fluid. The data can be accessed through a receiver or smartphone app.

3. Target Ranges:
Understanding your target blood sugar range is crucial for assessing your blood sugar levels. Target ranges can vary depending on factors such as age, medical

conditions, and individual circumstances. Consulting with a healthcare provider can help determine the appropriate target range for you. Generally, blood sugar targets aim for a balance between avoiding hypoglycemia (low blood sugar) and hyperglycemia (high blood sugar).

4. Patterns and Trends:
Assessing blood sugar levels involves looking for patterns and trends over time. This can help identify how specific foods, physical activity, stress, medication, and other factors influence your blood sugar levels. By observing patterns, you can make informed adjustments to your diet, exercise routine, and other lifestyle factors to better manage your blood sugar.

5. Glycated Hemoglobin (HbA1c) Test:
The HbA1c test gauges blood sugar levels on average during the previous two to three months. It provides a long-term picture of blood sugar control. This test assesses the

percentage of hemoglobin (a protein in red blood cells) that has sugar molecules attached to it. The result is expressed as a percentage, with lower percentages indicating better blood sugar control. The HbA1c test is typically conducted by a healthcare professional.

6. Record Keeping:
Keeping a record of your blood sugar levels, food intake, physical activity, medication, and other relevant factors can be helpful in assessing your blood sugar control. Maintaining a log or using smartphone apps designed for blood sugar tracking can provide valuable information to discuss with your healthcare provider and identify any necessary adjustments to your diabetes management plan.

Regularly assessing your blood sugar levels empowers you to take an active role in managing your health. It enables you to identify trends, make informed decisions, and work collaboratively with your healthcare team to optimize blood sugar control.

Identifying Signs of Blood Sugar Imbalance

It's essential to keep blood sugar levels steady for general health and wellbeing. When blood sugar levels become imbalanced, whether too high (hyperglycemia) or too low (hypoglycemia), it can have a significant impact on various bodily functions. Recognizing the signs of blood sugar imbalance is essential for prompt intervention and appropriate management. Here are common signs to watch for:

1. Symptoms of High Blood Sugar (Hyperglycemia):

- Frequent urination: Excess glucose in the bloodstream can lead to increased urination as the kidneys work to remove the excess sugar.
- Excessive thirst: Dehydration brought on by high blood sugar levels can result in excessive thirst.
- Fatigue and weakness: Cells may not effectively utilize glucose for energy, resulting in feelings of fatigue and weakness.
- Increased hunger: Despite high blood sugar levels, cells may not be receiving sufficient glucose, leading to persistent feelings of hunger.
- Blurred vision: High blood sugar can cause fluid to be drawn from the lenses of the eyes, affecting focus and resulting in blurred vision.
- Slow healing of wounds: Elevated blood sugar levels can impair the body's ability to heal wounds and recover from injuries.
- Recurrent infections: High blood sugar can weaken the immune system, making

individuals more susceptible to infections, particularly in the urinary tract, skin, and gums.
- Dry mouth and skin: High blood sugar can cause dehydration, leading to dry mouth and dry, itchy skin.
- Weight loss: Unexplained weight loss may occur due to the body's inability to utilize glucose efficiently.

2. Symptoms of Low Blood Sugar (Hypoglycemia):
- Shakiness and tremors: Hypoglycemia can cause trembling or shaking, especially in the hands.
- Sweating: Excessive sweating, particularly with cold and clammy skin, is a common symptom of low blood sugar.
- Rapid heartbeat: Hypoglycemia can trigger a rapid heartbeat or palpitations.
- Dizziness and lightheadedness: A feeling of dizziness or lightheadedness can occur when blood sugar levels drop too low.

- Irritability and mood changes: Hypoglycemia can affect mood, leading to irritability, anxiety, or even confusion.
- Hunger: Low blood sugar triggers hunger, often accompanied by intense cravings for sugary foods.
- Fatigue and weakness: Insufficient glucose in the bloodstream can result in feelings of fatigue, weakness, and difficulty concentrating.
- Headaches: Low blood sugar levels may cause headaches or migraines in some individuals.
- Blurred vision: Vision may become blurry, making it difficult to focus.

It is important to note that everyone's experience with blood sugar imbalance can vary, and symptoms may differ from person to person. If you suspect blood sugar imbalance, it is recommended to monitor your blood sugar levels using appropriate methods such as self-monitoring of blood glucose or continuous glucose monitoring devices.

If you experience persistent or severe symptoms of blood sugar imbalance, it is advisable to consult with a healthcare professional for further evaluation and guidance. They can provide an accurate diagnosis and help develop an appropriate management plan.

Common Risk Factors for Blood Sugar Dysregulation

Blood sugar dysregulation, including conditions like insulin resistance and diabetes, can result from a combination of genetic, lifestyle, and environmental factors. Understanding the common risk factors associated with blood sugar dysregulation is crucial for proactive management and prevention. The following are some important risk factors to be aware of:

1. Sedentary Lifestyle:
Leading a sedentary lifestyle, characterized by a lack of physical activity or prolonged periods of sitting, is a significant risk factor for blood sugar dysregulation. Regular exercise helps improve insulin sensitivity, allowing cells to effectively utilize glucose and maintain stable blood sugar levels.

2. Unhealthy Diet:
Consuming a diet high in processed foods, refined carbohydrates, added sugars, and unhealthy fats increases the risk of blood sugar dysregulation. These dietary decisions can result in weight gain, insulin resistance, and high blood sugar levels. A diet rich in whole foods, including fruits, vegetables, lean proteins, and whole grains, promotes stable blood sugar control.

3. Obesity or Excess Weight:

Excess weight, particularly abdominal obesity, significantly increases the risk of insulin resistance and blood sugar dysregulation. Adipose tissue, especially around the abdomen, produces hormones and substances that can interfere with insulin's actions, leading to elevated blood sugar levels.

4. Family History:
A family history of diabetes or blood sugar dysregulation increases an individual's risk. Genetic factors can contribute to impaired insulin production or reduced insulin sensitivity, making individuals more susceptible to blood sugar imbalances.

5. Age:
As individuals age, the risk of blood sugar dysregulation tends to increase. This is partly due to decreased physical activity levels, reduced muscle mass, and changes in hormonal regulation. However, blood sugar

dysregulation is not exclusive to older adults and can affect individuals of all age groups.

6. Gestational Diabetes:
Type 2 diabetes is more likely to occur in later life for women who had gestational diabetes during pregnancy. Additionally, the children born to mothers with gestational diabetes may have an increased risk of developing blood sugar dysregulation themselves.

7. Polycystic Ovary Syndrome (PCOS):
PCOS is a hormonal disorder that affects women and is characterized by irregular menstrual cycles, high levels of androgens (male hormones), and multiple ovarian cysts. Women with PCOS have an increased risk of insulin resistance and type 2 diabetes.

8. Certain Ethnic Backgrounds:
Certain ethnic backgrounds, such as African, Hispanic, Native American, Asian, and

Pacific Islander, have a higher predisposition to blood sugar dysregulation. These populations may be more susceptible to insulin resistance and an increased risk of developing diabetes.

9. Stress:
Chronic stress, whether related to work, personal life, or other factors, can impact blood sugar regulation. Stress hormones, such as cortisol, can raise blood sugar levels and contribute to insulin resistance over time.

10. Sleep Disorders:
Sleep disorders, including sleep apnea and insufficient sleep, can disrupt hormonal regulation and increase the risk of insulin resistance and blood sugar dysregulation.

Recognizing these common risk factors allows individuals to be proactive in managing their blood sugar levels. By addressing modifiable risk factors through lifestyle modifications, such as regular exercise, a balanced diet, stress management, and adequate sleep, individuals can reduce their risk of blood sugar dysregulation and associated health complications.

Diagnostic Tests for Assessing Blood Sugar Levels

When it comes to assessing blood sugar levels and determining the presence of blood sugar dysregulation, several diagnostic tests are available. These tests help healthcare professionals evaluate an individual's blood sugar control, diagnose conditions like diabetes or prediabetes, and monitor treatment effectiveness. Here are common diagnostic tests used to assess blood sugar levels:

1. Fasting Plasma Glucose (FPG) Test:

The fasting plasma glucose test measures blood sugar levels after an overnight fast of at least 8 hours. A blood sample is taken, and the glucose concentration in the plasma is measured. Diabetes is often indicated by FPG readings of 126 mg/dL or greater on two different occasions. FPG levels between 100 and 125 mg/dL may suggest prediabetes.

2. Oral Glucose Tolerance Test (OGTT): The oral glucose tolerance test is commonly used to diagnose gestational diabetes and evaluate blood sugar control in non-pregnant individuals. A fasting blood sample is obtained after an overnight fast. Then, the individual consumes a glucose-rich drink, and blood samples are taken at specific intervals over the next two hours to measure glucose levels. A blood sugar level of 200 mg/dL or higher at the two-hour mark typically indicates diabetes, while levels between 140 and 199 mg/dL may indicate prediabetes.

3. Hemoglobin A1c (HbA1c) Test:
The HbA1c test provides an indication of average blood sugar levels over the past two to three months. It measures the percentage of hemoglobin (a protein in red blood cells) that has sugar molecules attached to it. The result is expressed as a percentage. An HbA1c level of 6.5% or higher typically indicates diabetes, while levels between 5.7% and 6.4% may suggest prediabetes.

4. Random Plasma Glucose Test:
The random plasma glucose test involves measuring blood sugar levels at any time of the day, regardless of when the individual last ate. A random blood sample is taken, and a glucose level of 200 mg/dL or higher, along with symptoms of hyperglycemia, such as increased thirst or frequent urination, may indicate diabetes.

5. Continuous Glucose Monitoring (CGM):

Wearing a gadget that continuously monitors blood sugar levels day and night is known as continuous glucose monitoring. It provides real-time data, allowing individuals to track blood sugar patterns and trends. The interstitial fluid glucose levels are measured by CGM devices using a small sensor implanted beneath the skin. This method provides comprehensive information about blood sugar control over an extended period, helping individuals and healthcare professionals make informed decisions.

These diagnostic tests play a crucial role in assessing blood sugar levels, diagnosing diabetes or prediabetes, and monitoring treatment effectiveness. It is important to note that the interpretation of these tests should be done by a healthcare professional who can consider the individual's medical history, symptoms, and other factors.

Chapter 3

The Glucose Goddess Method Unveiled

"The Glucose Goddess Method" is a comprehensive and transformative approach to regulating blood sugar levels, improving health, and regaining stamina. Developed by leading experts in the field, this method combines scientific knowledge, practical strategies, and empowering techniques to help individuals achieve optimal blood sugar control and overall well-being. Let's delve into the key components and principles of The Glucose Goddess Method:

1. Holistic Approach:
The Glucose Goddess Method takes a holistic approach to blood sugar regulation, recognizing that various factors influence blood sugar levels and overall health. It goes

beyond diet and exercise, addressing lifestyle, stress management, sleep, emotional well-being, and other important aspects. This comprehensive approach ensures a well-rounded and sustainable path to blood sugar control.

2. Nutritional Guidance:
Proper nutrition plays a pivotal role in blood sugar regulation. The Glucose Goddess Method provides evidence-based nutritional guidance, focusing on whole, nutrient-dense foods that support stable blood sugar levels. It emphasizes the importance of balanced meals, portion control, mindful eating, and the inclusion of specific foods that promote optimal glucose metabolism.

3. Physical Activity and Exercise:
Regular physical activity and exercise are integral to blood sugar management. The Glucose Goddess Method incorporates personalized exercise recommendations, tailored to individual abilities and

preferences. It emphasizes the benefits of both aerobic exercise and strength training for improving insulin sensitivity, glucose utilization, and overall metabolic health.

4. Stress Management:
Chronic stress can contribute to blood sugar dysregulation. The Glucose Goddess Method recognizes the impact of stress on blood sugar control and provides practical strategies for stress reduction. Techniques such as mindfulness, meditation, deep breathing exercises, and lifestyle modifications are incorporated to help individuals manage stress effectively.

5. Sleep Optimization:
Quality sleep is essential for optimal blood sugar regulation. The Glucose Goddess Method emphasizes the importance of sleep hygiene and offers strategies to improve sleep quality and duration. Adequate sleep supports hormonal balance, insulin sensitivity, and overall metabolic health.

6. Mind-Body Connection:

The Glucose Goddess Method acknowledges the mind-body connection and the influence of emotions on blood sugar control. Techniques such as positive affirmations, visualization, and stress-reducing practices are integrated to promote emotional well-being and empower individuals in their blood sugar management journey.

7. Personalized Approach:

Every individual is unique, and their blood sugar management needs may vary. The Glucose Goddess Method embraces a personalized approach, taking into account individual circumstances, medical history, preferences, and goals. By tailoring the strategies and recommendations to each person's specific needs, it ensures a personalized and effective approach to blood sugar control.

8. Education and Empowerment:

Knowledge is empowering, and The Glucose Goddess Method provides individuals with the necessary education and resources to understand blood sugar regulation and its impact on overall health. It equips individuals with practical tools, tips, and actionable steps to take control of their blood sugar levels, make informed decisions, and achieve lasting results.

Principles and Philosophy of The Glucose Goddess Method

The Glucose Goddess Method is built upon a set of principles and a guiding philosophy that underpin its approach to blood sugar regulation and overall well-being. These principles form the foundation of the method and provide a framework for individuals to achieve optimal blood sugar control and transform their health. Let's explore the key principles and the underlying philosophy of The Glucose Goddess Method:

1. Balance and Moderation:
The Glucose Goddess Method promotes balance and moderation in all aspects of blood sugar regulation. It emphasizes the importance of balanced meals, incorporating a variety of nutrient-dense foods, and avoiding extremes or restrictive eating patterns. Balancing macronutrients, portion sizes, and meal timings helps maintain stable blood sugar levels and prevents excessive fluctuations.

2. Individualized Approach:
Recognizing that each person is unique, The Glucose Goddess Method takes an individualized approach to blood sugar management. It acknowledges that different factors, such as genetics, lifestyle, and preferences, can influence blood sugar control. By tailoring strategies and recommendations to each individual's

specific needs, the method ensures a personalized and effective approach to blood sugar regulation.

3. Empowerment and Education:
Education and empowerment are integral components of The Glucose Goddess Method. It aims to provide individuals with the knowledge and understanding they need to take control of their blood sugar levels and overall health. By empowering individuals with information, practical tools, and resources, the method enables them to make informed decisions and actively participate in their blood sugar management journey.

4. Sustainable Lifestyle Changes:
The Glucose Goddess Method promotes sustainable lifestyle changes that can be maintained in the long term. It emphasizes the adoption of healthy habits and gradual modifications to support blood sugar regulation and overall well-being. By

focusing on sustainable changes rather than short-term fixes, individuals can achieve lasting results and maintain optimal blood sugar control over time.

5. Mind-Body Connection:
The Glucose Goddess Method recognizes the interconnectedness of the mind and body in blood sugar regulation. It acknowledges the impact of stress, emotions, and mindset on blood sugar levels. By incorporating techniques such as stress management, mindfulness, and positive affirmations, the method addresses the mind-body connection and promotes emotional well-being alongside physical health.

6. Collaboration and Support:
Collaboration and support are central to The Glucose Goddess Method. It encourages individuals to work closely with healthcare professionals, such as doctors, dietitians, or diabetes educators, to receive personalized guidance and support. The method also

emphasizes the importance of seeking support from friends, family, or support groups, creating a community of like-minded individuals on the blood sugar management journey.

7. Continuous Learning and Adaptation: The Glucose Goddess Method values continuous learning and adaptation. It recognizes that the field of blood sugar regulation and health is constantly evolving, and new research and insights emerge over time. By staying open to new information and research, individuals can continue to refine their approach, adapt to new knowledge, and make adjustments to their blood sugar management strategies as needed.

The Glucose Goddess Method's philosophy revolves around empowering individuals to take control of their blood sugar levels and overall health. By embracing balance, individualization, education, sustainability, and the mind-body connection, individuals can embark on a transformative journey towards optimal blood sugar control, improved well-being, and a vibrant life.

Note: The term "Goddess" used in "The Glucose Goddess Method" is intended to be inclusive and empowering, representing the strength, power, and grace within individuals as they navigate their blood sugar management journey. It embraces a gender-neutral concept of empowerment and self-discovery.

Exploring the Four Pillars of Blood Sugar Balance

The Glucose Goddess Method is built upon the concept of four key pillars that form the foundation for achieving and maintaining optimal blood sugar balance. These pillars encompass various aspects of lifestyle, nutrition, and mindset, working together synergistically to support stable blood sugar levels. Let's delve into each of the four pillars and understand their significance:

1. Balanced Nutrition:
The first pillar focuses on nutrition and emphasizes the importance of consuming a balanced diet to support blood sugar balance. This involves incorporating a variety of whole, nutrient-dense foods, including lean proteins, complex carbohydrates, healthy fats, and fiber. The goal is to create balanced meals that provide sustained energy, promote satiety, and prevent rapid spikes or drops in blood sugar levels.

2. Regular Physical Activity:
Physical activity forms the second pillar of blood sugar balance. Engaging in regular exercise and physical activity helps improve insulin sensitivity, allowing the body to effectively utilize glucose for energy. Both

aerobic exercise and strength training have shown positive effects on blood sugar regulation. The Glucose Goddess Method encourages individuals to find physical activities they enjoy and incorporate them into their routine for optimal blood sugar control.

3. Stress Management:
Blood sugar levels can be significantly impacted by stress. The third pillar of blood sugar balance focuses on stress management techniques to promote emotional well-being and stable blood sugar control. Strategies such as mindfulness, deep breathing exercises, meditation, yoga, and adequate sleep play a crucial role in reducing stress and preventing stress-induced blood sugar imbalances.

4. Mindset and Mindfulness:
The fourth pillar centers around mindset and mindfulness, recognizing the powerful influence of thoughts and beliefs on blood

sugar regulation. Developing a positive mindset, cultivating self-compassion, and practicing mindful eating can help individuals make conscious food choices, tune into hunger and fullness cues, and develop a healthy relationship with food. By being present and mindful, individuals can make empowered decisions that support their blood sugar balance.

These four pillars of blood sugar balance work in harmony, reinforcing one another to create a comprehensive approach to blood sugar regulation and overall well-being. Each pillar is interconnected and equally important, contributing to stable blood sugar levels and improved health outcomes.

Strategies for Long-Term Success

Long-term success in blood sugar management requires a comprehensive and sustainable approach. The Glucose Goddess Method provides individuals with practical strategies that can be implemented over the long term, ensuring lasting results and improved overall health. Here are key strategies for achieving long-term success in blood sugar regulation:

1. Goal Setting and Tracking:
Setting clear, realistic goals is essential for long-term success. Define specific, measurable, achievable, relevant, and time-bound (SMART) goals that align with your blood sugar management journey. Whether it's reducing HbA1c levels, losing weight, or improving insulin sensitivity, having clear goals helps you stay focused and motivated. Regularly track your progress to celebrate milestones and make any necessary adjustments.

2. Meal Planning and Preparation:
Meal planning and preparation are powerful
tools for maintaining healthy eating habits
and blood sugar control. Plan your meals in
advance, incorporating a balance of
macronutrients and considering portion
sizes. Prepare meals and snacks in batches
to have healthy options readily available,
reducing the temptation to reach for
processed or high-sugar foods. Experiment
with new recipes and find enjoyment in
preparing nutritious meals that support
your blood sugar goals.

3. Portion Control and Mindful Eating:
Practicing portion control and mindful
eating can prevent overeating and support
stable blood sugar levels. Use smaller plates,
pay attention to portion sizes, and pay
attention to your body's signals of hunger
and fullness. Slow down while eating, savor
each bite, and pay attention to the taste,
texture, and satisfaction derived from your

meals. This mindful approach to eating can help you make healthier choices and avoid mindless snacking.

4. Regular Physical Activity:
Regular physical activity is a cornerstone of long-term success in blood sugar management. Find activities you like to do and incorporate them into your routine on a regular basis. Aim for a combination of aerobic exercises (such as walking, swimming, or cycling) and strength training to improve insulin sensitivity and support overall metabolic health. Strive for consistency rather than perfection, gradually increasing the duration and intensity of your workouts as you progress.

5. Stress Reduction Techniques:
Chronic stress can impact blood sugar control, so implementing stress reduction techniques is vital for long-term success. Find activities that help you unwind and manage stress effectively, such as yoga,

meditation, deep breathing exercises, or engaging in hobbies you enjoy. Prioritize self-care and create a supportive environment that fosters relaxation and emotional well-being.

6. Regular Monitoring and Follow-ups: Regular monitoring of your blood sugar levels is essential for maintaining long-term success. Work closely with healthcare professionals to track your progress and make any necessary adjustments to your treatment plan. Schedule regular follow-up appointments to discuss your blood sugar levels, address any concerns, and receive ongoing support and guidance.

7. Support System and Community: Building a support system and connecting with a community can greatly enhance your long-term success. Surround yourself with supportive family members, friends, or a support group who understand your goals and can provide encouragement and

accountability. Share your insights, look for counsel, and gain knowledge from those who are traveling a similar path.

8. Continuous Learning and Adaptation: Stay curious and open to continuous learning. Stay informed about new research, developments, and strategies related to blood sugar management. Be willing to adapt your approach as needed, considering individual responses and evolving circumstances. Continually seek knowledge and empower yourself with the latest information to optimize your blood sugar control.

By implementing these strategies for long-term success, you can create sustainable habits, maintain stable blood sugar levels, and improve your overall health and well-being.

Chapter 4

Nourishing Your Body for Optimal Blood Sugar Control

Proper nutrition plays a crucial role in achieving and maintaining optimal blood sugar control. The Glucose Goddess Method emphasizes the importance of nourishing your body with nutrient-dense foods that support stable blood sugar levels. By making mindful choices and adopting healthy eating habits, you can fuel your body effectively and support your blood sugar management goals. Here are key strategies for nourishing your body for optimal blood sugar control:

1. Embrace Whole, Unprocessed Foods: Focus on consuming whole, unprocessed foods that are rich in nutrients and minimally processed. These foods consist of fresh produce, entire grains, lean meats, and healthy fats. Whole foods provide a wide

array of vitamins, minerals, and fiber, supporting optimal blood sugar control and overall health.

2. Balance Macronutrients:
A balanced intake of macronutrients—carbohydrates, proteins, and fats—is essential for stable blood sugar levels. Aim for a well-rounded meal that includes all three macronutrients in appropriate proportions. Opt for complex carbohydrates that are slowly digested and provide a steady release of glucose into the bloodstream, such as whole grains, legumes, and vegetables. Combine carbohydrates with proteins and healthy fats to further slow down digestion and promote satiety.

3. Choose Low Glycemic Index Foods:
How quickly food-based carbs elevate blood sugar levels is gauged by the glycemic index (GI). Selecting foods with a lower GI can help prevent rapid spikes in blood sugar. Focus on incorporating low GI foods such as

non-starchy vegetables, whole grains, legumes, and most fruits. These foods are digested more slowly, leading to a gradual and steady release of glucose into the bloodstream.

4. Mindful Portion Control:
Be mindful of portion sizes to avoid overeating and excessive intake of carbohydrates. Use measuring cups, scales, or visual cues to understand appropriate portion sizes. Pay attention to your body's hunger and fullness cues, stopping eating when you feel comfortably satisfied. Mindful portion control ensures a balanced intake of nutrients and supports stable blood sugar levels.

5. Eat Regularly and Avoid Skipping Meals:
Maintaining a regular eating schedule and avoiding long gaps between meals is crucial for blood sugar control. Aim to eat meals and snacks at consistent intervals to provide a steady supply of glucose to your body.

Skipping meals or prolonged fasting can lead to imbalances in blood sugar levels. If you have specific dietary requirements or health conditions, work with a healthcare professional to determine the best meal timing for your needs.

6. Fiber-Rich Foods:
Include fiber-rich foods in your diet as they can help slow down the absorption of glucose, leading to more stable blood sugar levels. Foods such as whole grains, fruits, vegetables, legumes, and nuts are excellent sources of dietary fiber. Aim to incorporate a variety of these fiber-rich foods into your meals and snacks to support optimal blood sugar control and promote overall digestive health.

7. Hydration:
Staying hydrated is essential for overall health and blood sugar regulation. To stay well hydrated, consume enough water throughout the day. Limit the consumption

of sugary beverages and opt for water, herbal teas, or infused water instead. Proper hydration supports optimal cellular function and aids in the transportation of nutrients throughout the body.

8. Mindful Eating:
To develop a healthier connection with food, practice mindful eating. Slow down and savor each bite, paying attention to the flavors, textures, and sensations of the food. Avoid distractions while eating, such as watching TV or working on electronic devices. By being present and mindful during meals, you can better tune in to your body's hunger and fullness cues and make conscious choices that support your blood sugar control goals.

Nourishing your body with the right foods is a cornerstone of optimal blood sugar control. By incorporating whole, unprocessed foods, balancing macronutrients, choosing low GI foods, practicing portion control, and adopting mindful eating habits, you can provide your body with the nutrients it needs to maintain stable blood sugar levels and support overall well-being.

The Glucose Goddess Diet: Foods to Embrace and Avoid

The Glucose Goddess Method recognizes the importance of a balanced and nourishing diet for optimal blood sugar control. By embracing certain foods and avoiding others, you can support stable blood sugar levels and promote overall health. Here are the foods to embrace and avoid as part of The Glucose Goddess Diet:

Foods to Embrace:

1. Non-Starchy Vegetables:
Include a variety of non-starchy vegetables in your diet. These include leafy greens,

broccoli, cauliflower, peppers, cucumbers, zucchini, and asparagus. Non-starchy vegetables are low in carbohydrates and high in fiber, vitamins, and minerals, making them excellent choices for blood sugar control.

2. Whole Grains:
Select whole grains over refined grains, such as quinoa, brown rice, oats, and whole wheat bread. Fiber found in whole grains delays the absorption of glucose and supports stable blood sugar levels. They also provide essential nutrients and promote satiety.

3. Lean Proteins:
Incorporate lean protein sources into your meals, such as skinless poultry, fish, tofu, legumes, and low-fat dairy products. Protein helps stabilize blood sugar levels, promotes fullness, and supports muscle health. Choose lean cuts of meat and opt for

plant-based protein sources whenever possible.

4. Healthy Fats:
Include healthy fats in your diet, such as those found in salmon, avocados, nuts, seeds, and olive oil. Healthy fats provide satiety, support cardiovascular health, and help regulate blood sugar levels. However, since lipids are calorie-dense, portion control is crucial.

5. Low-Glycemic Fruits:
Select fruits with a lower glycemic index, such as berries, cherries, apples, pears, and citrus fruits. These fruits have less impact on blood sugar levels due to their fiber content. Enjoy them in moderation as part of a balanced meal or snack.

6. Legumes:
Legumes, including lentils, chickpeas, black beans, and kidney beans, are rich in fiber, protein, and complex carbohydrates. They

contribute to stable blood sugar levels, provide a feeling of fullness, and offer a variety of nutrients.

7. Herbs and Spices:
Enhance the flavor of your meals with herbs and spices like cinnamon, turmeric, ginger, garlic, and oregano. These seasonings not only add delicious taste but also have potential blood sugar-regulating properties.

Foods to Avoid or Limit:

1. Refined Sugars and Sweeteners:
Limit or avoid foods high in refined sugars and sweeteners, such as sugary beverages, candy, desserts, and processed snacks. These can cause rapid spikes in blood sugar levels and provide empty calories without essential nutrients.

2. Highly Processed Foods:
Reduce your intake of highly processed foods, including packaged snacks, fast food,

and pre-packaged meals. These often contain high levels of added sugars, unhealthy fats, and refined grains, which can negatively impact blood sugar control.

3. Sugary Beverages:
Drinks with added sugars should be avoided, such as soda, fruit juices, energy drinks, and sweetened teas. These can lead to a sudden surge in blood sugar levels due to their high sugar content. Instead, choose unsweetened beverages, water, or herbal tea.

4. Refined Grains:
Minimize consumption of refined grains such as white bread, white rice, and sugary cereals. These foods have had their fiber and nutrients removed, leading to a quicker spike in blood sugar levels compared to whole grains.

5. Saturated and Trans Fats:

Limit intake of saturated and trans fats found in fried foods, fatty cuts of meat, processed snacks, and baked goods. These fats can contribute to insulin resistance and increase the risk of cardiovascular disease.

6. Excessive Alcohol:
Moderate alcohol consumption is recommended, but excessive intake can disrupt blood sugar regulation. Limit alcohol consumption and be mindful of its effects on blood sugar levels.

Remember, individual needs and responses may vary. It's important to consult with a healthcare professional or registered dietitian to personalize your diet and ensure it aligns with your specific health needs and goals.

Meal Preparation and Portion Control for Blood Sugar Stability

Meal planning and portion control are essential components of achieving stable blood sugar levels. By carefully considering the foods you eat, their portion sizes, and their distribution throughout the day, you can support optimal blood sugar control and promote overall health. Here are key strategies for effective meal planning and portion control:

1. Balance Macronutrients:
Each meal should consist of a balance of macronutrients: carbohydrates, proteins, and fats. Including all three macronutrients in appropriate proportions helps slow down the absorption of glucose and promotes stable blood sugar levels. Aim for a plate that is roughly divided into thirds, with one-third dedicated to lean protein, one-third to non-starchy vegetables, and one-third to whole grains or other complex

carbohydrates, combined with a tiny amount of good fats.

2. Choose Complex Carbohydrates:
Focus on incorporating complex carbohydrates into your meals. These carbohydrates, found in whole grains, legumes, and starchy vegetables, are digested more slowly, resulting in a gradual and steady release of glucose into the bloodstream. This helps prevent rapid spikes in blood sugar levels. Opt for brown rice, quinoa, whole wheat bread, sweet potatoes, and beans as sources of complex carbohydrates.

3. Fiber-Rich Foods:
Include fiber-rich foods in your meals. Fiber slows down digestion, helps control blood sugar levels, and promotes a feeling of fullness. Non-starchy vegetables, fruits, whole grains, legumes, and nuts are excellent sources of dietary fiber.

Incorporate as many of these foods as you can into your meals and snacks.

4. Mindful Portion Control:
Be mindful of portion sizes to avoid overeating and excessive carbohydrate intake. Use measuring cups, scales, or visual cues to understand appropriate portion sizes. Remember that portion control is not only about carbohydrates but also about proteins and fats. Consider using smaller plates and bowls to help manage portion sizes visually.

5. Regular Meal Times and Frequency:
Maintaining regular meal times and spacing meals evenly throughout the day helps promote stable blood sugar levels. Aim for three main meals (breakfast, lunch, and dinner) and include snacks if needed, such as a mid-morning and mid-afternoon snack. Avoid prolonged periods without eating to

prevent blood sugar fluctuations. However, individual needs may vary, so work with a healthcare professional to determine the meal timing that suits you best.

6. Snack Smartly:
Choose healthy, balanced snacks that provide a combination of macronutrients and contribute to stable blood sugar levels. Opt for snacks such as Greek yogurt with berries, a handful of nuts, sliced vegetables with hummus, or a small apple with almond butter. Avoid sugary snacks and processed foods that can lead to rapid blood sugar spikes.

7. Hydration:
Drink enough water to keep yourself hydrated all day long. Proper hydration supports overall health and can help maintain optimal blood sugar control. Limit or avoid sugary beverages, as they can contribute to blood sugar imbalances.

8. Monitor and Adjust:
Regularly monitor your blood sugar levels and adjust your meal planning and portion sizes accordingly. Work closely with your healthcare professional to understand your target blood sugar ranges and adjust your diet as needed. This will help ensure that your meal plan is personalized and effective for your individual needs.

Superfoods and Supplements for Blood Sugar Support

In addition to a well-balanced diet, certain superfoods and supplements can provide additional support for maintaining stable blood sugar levels. These nutrient-dense foods and supplements contain specific compounds that have shown potential in supporting blood sugar regulation and overall health. Here are some superfoods and supplements that you may consider incorporating into your routine:

1. Cinnamon:
Cinnamon is a spice with potential blood sugar-lowering effects. It may improve insulin sensitivity, enhance glucose metabolism, and reduce post-meal blood sugar spikes. Add cinnamon to your meals, such as sprinkling it on oatmeal, yogurt, or incorporating it into homemade smoothies or baked goods.

2. Berries:
Berries, such as blueberries, strawberries, and raspberries, are rich in antioxidants, fiber, and polyphenols. They have a low glycemic index and may help regulate blood sugar levels. Enjoy a handful of fresh berries as a snack, or add them to smoothies, yogurt, or salads.

3. Turmeric:

A substance found in turmeric called curcumin has both anti-inflammatory and antioxidant effects. Some studies suggest that curcumin may improve insulin sensitivity and help manage blood sugar levels. Incorporate turmeric into your cooking or consider taking a curcumin supplement, following the recommended dosage.

4. Green Leafy Vegetables:
Green leafy vegetables, including spinach, kale, and Swiss chard, are packed with nutrients, including magnesium, which plays a role in glucose metabolism and insulin sensitivity. Add a generous portion of leafy greens to your salads, stir-fries, or smoothies.

5. Omega-3 Fatty Acids:
Omega-3 fatty acids, found in fatty fish like salmon, mackerel, and sardines, as well as in chia seeds and flaxseeds, have anti-inflammatory properties and may

support blood sugar control. Aim to incorporate omega-3-rich foods into your diet regularly. If needed, you can also consider a high-quality fish oil or algae-based omega-3 supplement.

6. Chromium:
Mineral chromium is involved in the metabolism of lipids and carbohydrates. It may enhance insulin sensitivity and help regulate blood sugar levels. Good food sources of chromium include broccoli, green beans, nuts, and whole grains. Consult with a healthcare professional to determine if a chromium supplement is appropriate for you.

7. Magnesium:
Magnesium is an essential mineral involved in various enzymatic reactions, including those related to glucose metabolism. It may help improve insulin sensitivity and support stable blood sugar levels. Magnesium-rich foods include almonds, spinach, avocados,

and dark chocolate. You can also discuss magnesium supplementation with your healthcare professional if needed.

8. Probiotics:
Probiotics are beneficial bacteria that promote gut health and may play a role in blood sugar regulation. They are present in fermented foods like kimchi, sauerkraut, kefir, and yogurt. Consider incorporating these foods into your diet or discuss a high-quality probiotic supplement with your healthcare professional.

While superfoods and supplements can provide additional support, it's important to remember that they should complement a healthy diet and lifestyle. It's always advisable to consult with a healthcare professional or registered dietitian before starting any new supplements to ensure they are suitable for your individual needs, especially if you take medication or have underlying health issues.

Incorporating these superfoods and supplements, along with a balanced diet and regular exercise, can contribute to better blood sugar control and overall well-being. Remember to focus on whole, nutrient-dense foods as the foundation of your blood sugar management strategy.

Chapter 5

Exercise and Blood Sugar Regulation

Regular physical activity and exercise play a crucial role in blood sugar regulation and overall health. Exercise helps improve insulin sensitivity, enhances glucose uptake by muscles, and promotes the efficient use of glucose for energy. Here's how exercise can positively impact blood sugar regulation:

1. Increased Insulin Sensitivity:
Exercise improves insulin sensitivity, allowing your cells to more effectively use insulin to transport glucose from the bloodstream into the cells. This helps maintain stable blood sugar levels and reduces the risk of insulin resistance.

2. Glucose Uptake by Muscles:

During exercise, muscles become more responsive to insulin, allowing them to take up glucose from the bloodstream without relying heavily on insulin. This process helps lower blood sugar levels and promotes the efficient use of glucose for energy.

3. Improved Glucose Control:
Engaging in regular physical activity helps regulate blood sugar levels by utilizing excess glucose stored in the muscles and liver as glycogen. This mechanism helps prevent sharp increases in blood sugar after meals and supports more stable levels throughout the day.

4. Weight Management:
Exercise contributes to weight management and can help prevent or manage obesity, a risk factor for blood sugar dysregulation. Maintaining a healthy weight through regular physical activity can enhance insulin sensitivity and reduce the risk of developing type 2 diabetes.

5. Reduced Insulin Resistance:
Regular exercise reduces insulin resistance,
a condition in which cells become less
responsive to insulin. By reducing insulin
resistance, exercise helps improve blood
sugar control and lowers the risk of type 2
diabetes.

6. Post-Exercise Blood Sugar Benefits:
Exercise can have a positive impact on blood
sugar levels even after the activity is
completed. After exercise, your body
continues to use glucose for energy, which
can help lower blood sugar levels for hours
following the workout.

7. Stress Reduction:
Engaging in physical activity also helps
reduce stress levels, which can indirectly
contribute to better blood sugar control.
Chronic stress can lead to elevated blood
sugar levels, so incorporating exercise as a
stress management tool can be beneficial.

8. Cardiovascular Health:
Regular exercise promotes cardiovascular
health, reducing the risk of heart disease
and related complications that can arise
from uncontrolled blood sugar levels. It
supports healthy blood pressure, cholesterol
levels, and overall heart function.

It's important to note that individuals with
diabetes or other medical conditions should
consult with their healthcare professional
before starting or modifying an exercise
routine. Your healthcare provider can
provide personalized guidance on the type,
intensity, and duration of exercise that best
suits your needs and health status.

In conclusion, incorporating regular
exercise into your lifestyle can significantly
contribute to blood sugar regulation and
overall well-being. Whether it's aerobic
activities like brisk walking, running,
swimming, or cycling, or strength training

exercises, finding enjoyable forms of physical activity can help you maintain stable blood sugar levels, improve insulin sensitivity, and support your overall health.

Tailoring Your Workout Routine for Maximum Benefits

Designing a workout routine that is tailored to your needs and goals is essential for maximizing the benefits of exercise. Whether you're aiming to balance blood sugar levels, improve overall fitness, or achieve specific health outcomes, customizing your workout routine can help you reach your desired results more effectively. Here are some key considerations for tailoring your workout routine for maximum benefits:

1. Consult with a Healthcare Professional: Before starting or modifying any exercise routine, it is crucial to consult with a healthcare professional, especially if you

have underlying health conditions or concerns. They can provide guidance based on your medical history, current fitness level, and specific goals, ensuring that your workout routine is safe and suitable for your individual needs.

2. Set Clear Goals:
Identify your specific fitness or health goals. Are you primarily focused on blood sugar regulation, weight management, cardiovascular health, strength improvement, or a combination of these? Setting clear goals will help you choose the appropriate types of exercises and create a well-rounded routine.

3. Incorporate Aerobic Exercise:
Aerobic exercises, also known as cardiovascular exercises, increase heart rate and breathing rate, improving cardiovascular health and assisting in weight management. Choose activities you enjoy, such as brisk walking, jogging,

cycling, swimming, or aerobic classes. Aim for 75 minutes of strenuous activity scattered throughout the week, or at least 150 minutes of moderate aerobic activity every week.

4. Include Strength Training:
Strength training exercises help build and maintain muscle mass, improve bone density, and enhance overall strength and stability. Incorporate resistance training exercises using weights, resistance bands, or bodyweight exercises like push-ups, squats, and lunges. Aim for at least two to three sessions per week, targeting major muscle groups with 8-12 repetitions of each exercise.

5. Prioritize Interval Training:
Interval training, which involves alternating between high-intensity bursts of exercise and lower-intensity recovery periods, can be particularly beneficial for blood sugar regulation. High-intensity interval training

(HIIT) has been shown to improve insulin sensitivity and glucose metabolism. Include short bursts of intense exercise, such as sprint intervals or circuit training, in your routine. Start gradually and increase the intensity as your fitness level improves.

6. Consider Flexibility and Balance Exercises:
Include flexibility and balance exercises to improve mobility, reduce the risk of injuries, and enhance overall fitness. Incorporate activities like yoga, Pilates, tai chi, or stretching exercises. These exercises can help with stress reduction and promote relaxation, which may indirectly contribute to better blood sugar control.

7. Monitor Intensity:
Pay attention to the intensity of your workouts. Monitoring your heart rate, perceived exertion, or using wearable fitness trackers can help ensure that you are working at an appropriate level. Work

within your comfort range while continuing to push yourself. Gradually progress your intensity over time as your fitness improves.

8. Stay Consistent:
Consistency is key for achieving maximum benefits from your workout routine. Aim for regular exercise sessions throughout the week, rather than sporadic bursts of activity. Find a schedule that works for you and make exercise a priority in your daily life.

9. Listen to Your Body:
Be mindful of your body's signals and adjust your routine accordingly. If you experience any discomfort or pain during exercise, modify or seek guidance from a professional. Rest and recovery are equally important for allowing your body to adapt and reap the benefits of your workouts.

Remember, it's important to personalize your workout routine based on your individual needs, preferences, and fitness level. Gradually progress the intensity and duration of your workouts to avoid overexertion and reduce the risk of injuries. By tailoring your workout routine to your goals and capabilities, you can optimize the benefits of exercise, including blood sugar regulation, overall fitness, and improved well-being.

Combining Cardiovascular and Strength Training for Stamina

When it comes to building stamina, combining cardiovascular exercise with strength training can be a powerful approach. Cardiovascular exercise improves your heart health, lung capacity, and endurance, while strength training enhances your muscle strength, power, and overall physical resilience. By incorporating both types of exercise into your routine, you can maximize your stamina and achieve better overall fitness. Here's how to combine cardiovascular and strength training for stamina:

1. Start with Cardiovascular Exercise: Begin your workout with cardiovascular exercise to warm up your body, increase your heart rate, and improve blood flow. Choose activities that raise your heart rate and challenge your cardiovascular system, such as jogging, cycling, swimming, or using a cardio machine like a treadmill or elliptical trainer. Aim for a moderate intensity level that allows you to maintain a conversation but still feel exerted.

2. Alternate Between Cardio and Strength Training Sets: After your warm-up, incorporate strength training exercises into your routine. Alternate between cardiovascular exercises and strength training sets to create a well-rounded workout. For example,

perform a set of strength exercises targeting different muscle groups, such as squats, push-ups, lunges, or dumbbell curls, followed by a few minutes of cardiovascular exercise like jumping jacks or jogging in place. Repeat this pattern throughout your workout session.

3. Choose Compound Exercises:
Opt for compound exercises that engage multiple muscle groups simultaneously during your strength training sets. These exercises are more effective at building overall strength and stamina. Examples include squats, deadlifts, bench presses, rows, and overhead presses. Compound exercises require more energy and increase your heart rate, contributing to cardiovascular conditioning alongside strength development.

4. Incorporate High-Intensity Interval Training (HIIT):

Integrate high-intensity interval training (HIIT) into your cardiovascular workouts to boost stamina. HIIT involves alternating between short bursts of intense exercise and active recovery periods. For instance, sprint for 30 seconds, followed by a 1-minute recovery period of light jogging or walking. Repeat this cycle several times during your cardio session. HIIT is highly effective for improving cardiovascular fitness and increasing endurance.

5. Focus on Endurance and Repetitions: When strength training, emphasize higher repetitions with moderate weights or bodyweight exercises to build endurance. This approach helps condition your muscles to sustain effort over an extended period. For example, perform three sets of 12-15 repetitions per exercise. Gradually increase the resistance or intensity as your stamina improves.

6. Include Circuit Training:

Incorporate circuit training into your workout routine. Circuit training involves performing a series of exercises consecutively, targeting different muscle groups, with minimal rest in between. This method keeps your heart rate elevated throughout the session, combining strength training and cardiovascular benefits. Customize your circuit by selecting a mix of compound exercises, bodyweight movements, and cardiovascular exercises.

7. Pay Attention to Recovery:
Allow sufficient time for rest and recovery between sets and workouts. Adequate rest is crucial for your muscles to recover, repair, and grow stronger. Overtraining can lead to fatigue, decreased stamina, and increased risk of injury. Aim for at least one or two rest days per week and consider incorporating activities like yoga, stretching, or low-impact activities on your recovery days.

8. Progress Gradually:

To continually improve stamina, gradually increase the duration, intensity, or complexity of your workouts. Gradual progression challenges your body, helping it adapt and become more resilient over time. Monitor your progress, and when exercises become too easy, increase weights, add more repetitions, or try more advanced variations to continue challenging yourself.

Chapter 6

Stress Management Techniques for Blood Sugar Control

Managing stress is essential for maintaining stable blood sugar levels. When you experience stress, your body releases hormones that can raise blood sugar levels and disrupt the balance of glucose regulation. Incorporating stress management techniques into your daily routine can help you reduce stress levels and improve blood sugar control. Here are some effective techniques for managing stress:

1. Deep Breathing and Relaxation Exercises: Exercises that involve deep breathing can trigger the body's relaxation response, which lowers tension and fosters a sense of peace. Practice deep abdominal breathing

by inhaling deeply through your nose, expanding your abdomen, and exhaling slowly through your mouth. Combine deep breathing with relaxation exercises like progressive muscle relaxation or guided imagery to further enhance the relaxation response.

2. Mindfulness and Meditation:
Meditation and mindfulness exercises can lower stress and enhance general wellbeing. Being mindful means paying close attention to the here and now without passing judgment. This can be done through mindful breathing, body scans, or mindful walking. Meditation techniques, such as mindfulness meditation or loving-kindness meditation, can also promote relaxation and reduce stress levels.

3. Regular Physical Activity:
Regular physical activity not only improves physical health but also lowers stress levels. Exercise causes the body to release

endorphins, which are naturally uplifting substances. Find activities that you enjoy, such as walking, jogging, yoga, or dancing, and aim for at least 30 minutes of moderate-intensity exercise most days of the week.

4. Social Support:
Maintaining strong social connections and seeking support from friends, family, or support groups can help alleviate stress. Talking to someone you trust about your concerns and feelings can provide emotional support and different perspectives. Engaging in social activities and fostering positive relationships can also contribute to a sense of well-being and stress reduction.

5. Time Management and Prioritization:
Organizing your time effectively and setting priorities can reduce feelings of overwhelm and stress. Break tasks into smaller, manageable steps, and create a realistic schedule. Prioritize important activities and

delegate tasks when possible. Setting boundaries and learning to say no to excessive commitments can also help reduce stress levels.

6. Healthy Lifestyle Choices:
Maintaining a healthy lifestyle can contribute to stress reduction and better blood sugar control. Ensure you're getting enough sleep, as lack of sleep can increase stress levels. Eat a balanced diet rich in whole foods, including fruits, vegetables, lean proteins, and whole grains. Limit your intake of processed foods, sugary snacks, and caffeine, as they can contribute to blood sugar fluctuations and increased stress.

7. Relaxation Techniques:
Incorporate relaxation techniques into your daily routine to reduce stress. Examples include listening to calming music, practicing yoga or tai chi, taking warm baths, or engaging in hobbies that promote relaxation, such as reading, gardening, or

painting. Find activities that help you unwind and make time for them regularly.

8. Cognitive-Behavioral Techniques:
Cognitive-behavioral techniques can help manage stress by identifying and modifying negative thought patterns. Practice reframing negative thoughts into more positive and realistic ones. Challenge irrational beliefs and practice self-compassion. Engaging in cognitive-behavioral therapy or working with a therapist can provide additional support and guidance.

9. Prioritize Self-Care:
Make self-care a priority in your daily life. Take part in things that make you happy, content, and relaxed. This can include hobbies, self-reflection, spending time in nature, or engaging in creative pursuits. Taking care of your emotional, physical, and mental well-being is crucial for managing stress and promoting blood sugar control.

Remember, finding the right stress management techniques may require some trial and error. Experiment with different techniques and discover what works best for you.

Recognizing the Relationship between Stress and Blood Sugar

The relationship between stress and blood sugar levels is intricate and multifaceted. When you experience stress, whether it's due to physical, emotional, or environmental factors, your body responds by releasing stress hormones such as cortisol and adrenaline. These hormones trigger a series of physiological responses, including an increase in blood sugar levels. Here's a closer look at the connection between stress and blood sugar:

1. Stress Hormones and Glucose Release:
Stress hormones, particularly cortisol, have a direct impact on glucose metabolism. They stimulate the liver to release stored glucose into the bloodstream, providing an energy boost in response to perceived threats. This glucose release is part of the body's natural "fight-or-flight" response designed to help you cope with stress.

2. Insulin Resistance:
Prolonged or chronic stress can lead to insulin resistance. When stress hormones are constantly elevated, cells may become less responsive to the effects of insulin, the hormone responsible for regulating blood sugar. Insulin resistance makes it more difficult for glucose to enter the cells, resulting in higher blood sugar levels.

3. Emotional Eating and Cravings:
Stress can influence eating behaviors and lead to emotional eating or cravings for high-calorie, sugary foods. This response is

partly due to the release of stress hormones, which can trigger the brain's reward system and increase the desire for comfort foods. Consuming these foods can cause rapid spikes in blood sugar levels.

4. Disrupted Meal Patterns and Poor Food Choices:
During periods of stress, individuals may experience disruptions in their regular meal patterns. They may skip meals or opt for quick, convenient, and often unhealthy food choices. These dietary changes, combined with stress-induced hormonal fluctuations, can contribute to unstable blood sugar levels.

5. Impaired Sleep:
Stress can negatively impact sleep quality and duration. Lack of sleep or poor sleep quality has been associated with increased stress levels and disturbances in glucose metabolism. Inadequate sleep can affect

insulin sensitivity and lead to higher blood sugar levels.

6. Impact on Self-Care Practices:
Stress can also influence self-care practices such as exercise, meal planning, and stress management techniques. When stressed, individuals may neglect these healthy behaviors, further contributing to blood sugar imbalances.

7. Vicious Cycle:
The relationship between stress and blood sugar forms a vicious cycle. High stress levels can lead to elevated blood sugar, and increased blood sugar levels can, in turn, contribute to feelings of stress and anxiety. This cycle can be challenging to break without implementing effective stress management strategies.

Understanding the connection between stress and blood sugar is crucial for individuals looking to manage their blood sugar levels effectively. By managing stress levels, individuals can support better glucose regulation and overall well-being. Implementing stress management techniques, adopting healthy lifestyle habits, and seeking support when needed can help break the cycle and promote stable blood sugar control.

Implementing Relaxation and Mindfulness Practices

Relaxation and mindfulness practices can be powerful tools for managing stress, promoting emotional well-being, and supporting stable blood sugar control. By incorporating these practices into your daily routine, you can cultivate a sense of calm, reduce stress levels, and enhance your overall health. Here are some effective relaxation and mindfulness techniques to consider:

1. Deep Breathing:
Deep breathing exercises can instantly induce a state of relaxation. Find a quiet and comfortable space. Take slow, deep breaths, inhaling deeply through your nose, filling your abdomen with air, and exhaling slowly through your mouth. Focus your attention on the sensation of your breath, letting go of any tension or stress with each exhale.

2. Progressive Muscle Relaxation:
Progressive muscle relaxation involves systematically tensing and releasing different muscle groups to promote physical and mental relaxation. Start from your toes and work your way up to your head, tensing each muscle group for a few seconds and then releasing the tension. Pay attention to the sensations of relaxation and relief as you let go of muscle tension.

3. Mindful Meditation:

Mindful meditation involves bringing your attention to the present moment without judgment. Find a quiet and comfortable space, sit or lie down, and focus on your breath, bodily sensations, or a specific object of your choosing. Whenever your mind wanders, gently bring your attention back to your chosen focal point, practicing non-judgment and acceptance of your thoughts and feelings.

4. Guided Imagery:
Guided imagery involves using your imagination to create calming mental images or scenes. Close your eyes and picture a tranquil setting, such a beach or a forest. Engage all your senses by imagining the sights, sounds, smells, and sensations of this place. Allow yourself to immerse in the experience and let go of stress as you engage with your imagination.

5. Mindful Eating:

Mindful eating involves bringing full awareness to the process of eating, paying attention to the sensory experiences, and savoring each bite. Engage your senses by noticing the colors, textures, and flavors of your food. Eat slowly and chew your food thoroughly. Be present and non-judgmental about your eating experience, focusing on nourishing your body and enjoying the moment.

6. Nature Connection:
The mind and body can be calmed and rejuvenated by spending time in nature. Go for a stroll in a park, garden, or other natural setting. Pay close attention to the natural world's noises, sights, and sensations. Breathe deeply and take in the peace and beauty that surrounds you. Connecting with nature can help reduce stress and promote a sense of well-being.

7. Gratitude Practice:

Practicing gratitude involves consciously focusing on the things you are grateful for in your life. Regularly take a few moments to reflect on and write down the things you appreciate. It can be as simple as a beautiful sunrise, a supportive friend, or a good meal. Cultivating gratitude shifts your focus to positive aspects of your life and promotes a more positive outlook.

8. Mindful Movement:
Engaging in mindful movement practices, such as yoga, tai chi, or qigong, can help promote relaxation, improve flexibility, and reduce stress. These practices combine gentle movements with breath awareness, promoting a mind-body connection and a sense of inner calm.

Remember, relaxation and mindfulness practices are personal and can be tailored to suit your preferences and needs.

Strategies for Better Sleep and Hormonal Balance

Getting quality sleep is vital for maintaining hormonal balance, overall health, and stable blood sugar levels. Sleep plays a crucial role in regulating hormones involved in glucose metabolism, appetite control, and stress response. Implementing effective strategies for better sleep can contribute to improved hormonal balance. Here are some strategies to consider:

1. Establish a Consistent Sleep Schedule: Even on weekends, have a consistent sleep routine by going to bed and waking up at the same time every day. This encourages a more regular sleep-wake cycle and assists in regulating your body's internal clock.

2. Create a Relaxing Bedtime Routine: Create a calming ritual before bed to tell your body it's time to relax. You could do things like read a book, take a warm bath,

practice relaxation techniques, or listen to relaxing music as a way to do this. When it's almost time for bed, stay away from stimulating activities and bright devices because they can disrupt sleep.

3. Create a Sleep-Friendly Environment: Optimize your sleep environment for comfort and relaxation. Keep your bedroom cool, dark, and quiet. Use blackout curtains or an eye mask to block out light, earplugs or white noise machines to reduce noise disruptions, and a comfortable mattress and pillows that support good sleep posture.

4. Limit Exposure to Electronic Devices: Your body's regular sleep-wake cycle may be hampered by the blue light that electronic gadgets like computers, tablets, and smartphones emit. Avoid using these devices for at least an hour before bed. If necessary, use blue light-blocking glasses or

enable the night mode on your devices to reduce exposure.

5. Create a Calming Bedroom Environment:
Use aromatherapy, such as lavender essential oil, to create a calming atmosphere in your bedroom. The scent of lavender has been shown to promote relaxation and better sleep quality. You can put a few drops on your pillow or use an essential oil diffuser.

6. Regular Physical Activity:
Regular physical activity during the day can help you sleep better at night. On most days of the week, try to get in at least 30 minutes of moderate activity. However, avoid exercising too close to bedtime, as it may energize your body and make it difficult to fall asleep.

7. Limit Stimulants and Alcohol:
Reduce or eliminate the consumption of stimulants like caffeine and nicotine,

particularly in the afternoon and evening. These substances can interfere with your ability to fall asleep and maintain quality sleep. Additionally, while alcohol may initially make you feel drowsy, it can disrupt the deeper stages of sleep and lead to restless nights.

8. Manage Stress:
Stress can significantly impact sleep quality and hormonal balance. Implement stress management techniques such as deep breathing, meditation, or journaling before bed to help calm the mind and reduce stress levels. Engaging in regular exercise, maintaining a balanced lifestyle, and seeking support from friends, family, or a therapist can also help manage stress effectively.

9. Create a Comfortable Sleep Environment:
Invest in a comfortable mattress, pillows, and bedding that suit your individual needs and preferences. Ensure your bedroom is

adequately ventilated, at a temperature that promotes restful sleep (usually between 60-67°F or 15-19°C), and free from distractions that may disturb your sleep.

10. Seek Professional Guidance:
If you constantly struggle with sleep issues or suspect an underlying sleep disorder, consider consulting a healthcare professional or a sleep specialist. They can provide a comprehensive evaluation, diagnosis, and recommend appropriate treatments or therapies.

Remember, everyone's sleep needs may vary, so it's essential to listen to your body and adjust your sleep routine accordingly. By prioritizing quality sleep, you support hormonal balance, enhance overall well-being, and optimize blood sugar control.

Chapter 7

Tracking and Monitoring Your Progress

Tracking and monitoring your progress is an essential aspect of the Glucose Goddess Method. It allows you to assess your journey towards blood sugar regulation, improved health, and increased stamina. By keeping track of key indicators, you can gain valuable insights, identify patterns, and make informed adjustments to your approach. Here are some strategies for effectively tracking and monitoring your progress:

1. Blood Sugar Monitoring:
Regularly monitor your blood sugar levels using a glucose meter or continuous glucose monitor (CGM). Follow the recommended testing frequency advised by your healthcare provider and record your results in a

logbook or a digital tracking tool. This data will help you identify trends, understand how different foods and activities affect your blood sugar levels, and make necessary adjustments to your diet and lifestyle.

2. Food Diary:
Keep a detailed food diary to track your dietary intake. Record what you eat and drink throughout the day, including portion sizes and meal timings. Note any symptoms or changes in blood sugar levels after consuming specific foods or meals. This information will help you identify foods that may cause blood sugar imbalances and make more informed choices for optimal blood sugar control.

3. Physical Activity Log:
Maintain a physical activity log to track your exercise routines, including the type, duration, and intensity of each activity. Note how exercise impacts your blood sugar levels, energy levels, and overall well-being.

This log will enable you to monitor your fitness progress and adjust your workouts for maximum benefits and blood sugar regulation.

4. Symptom Journal:
Keep a journal to track any symptoms or changes you experience related to blood sugar regulation. Note any signs of high or low blood sugar, such as fatigue, increased thirst, frequent urination, or mood swings. By documenting these symptoms, you can identify triggers, patterns, and potential areas for improvement in your routine.

5. Measurements and Body Metrics:
Take regular measurements of your weight, waist circumference, and other relevant body metrics. These measurements can serve as additional markers of progress and help you track changes in body composition and overall health. However, remember that progress is not solely defined by numbers on

a scale but also by improvements in energy levels, well-being, and blood sugar control.

6. Reflection and Self-Assessment:
Set aside time regularly to reflect on your progress, challenges, and achievements. Consider how your blood sugar levels, overall health, and stamina have improved since implementing the Glucose Goddess Method. Assess the effectiveness of the strategies you've implemented and identify areas where you can make further adjustments or seek additional support.

7. Regular Check-Ins with Healthcare Provider:
Schedule regular check-ins with your healthcare provider, such as a doctor, nutritionist, or diabetes educator. Share your tracking data, including blood sugar logs, food diary, and physical activity logs. Discuss any concerns, questions, or challenges you may be facing. Your healthcare provider can provide guidance,

offer personalized recommendations, and monitor your progress from a medical perspective.

8. Celebrate Milestones and Achievements: Celebrate your progress along the journey and your milestones.Recognize the positive changes you've made, whether they are improvements in blood sugar control, weight loss, increased energy, or better overall well-being. Celebrating these achievements can help maintain motivation and reinforce healthy habits.

Remember, tracking and monitoring your progress is not about perfection but rather about gaining insights, making informed decisions, and adjusting your approach as needed. It's a valuable tool in understanding how your body responds to various factors and guiding you towards optimal blood sugar regulation, improved health, and increased stamina.

Tools and Techniques for Monitoring Blood Sugar Levels

Monitoring blood sugar levels is a fundamental aspect of managing blood sugar regulation and the Glucose Goddess Method. Regular monitoring helps you understand how your body responds to different foods, activities, and medications, allowing you to make informed decisions for optimal blood sugar control. Here are some tools and techniques for monitoring your blood sugar levels effectively:

1. Glucose Meters:
Glucose meters are portable devices that measure your blood sugar levels. They require a small blood sample obtained by pricking your finger with a lancet. Follow the instructions provided with your meter to obtain accurate readings. Some meters also

offer features like memory storage, data tracking, and the ability to calculate averages over time.

2. Continuous Glucose Monitoring (CGM) Systems:

CGM systems provide continuous real-time monitoring of your blood sugar levels. These systems consist of a small sensor inserted under your skin, typically on the abdomen or arm, and a receiver or smartphone app that displays your glucose readings. CGMs offer valuable insights into glucose patterns throughout the day, including trends, highs, lows, and the impact of meals and activities.

3. Flash Glucose Monitoring (FGM) Systems:

FGM systems, such as FreeStyle Libre, are similar to CGMs but do not provide real-time glucose readings. Instead, you use a reader or smartphone app to scan a sensor worn on your skin to obtain glucose readings. FGM systems offer the convenience of obtaining glucose information without the need for routine finger pricks.

4. Mobile Apps and Digital Platforms:
There are numerous mobile apps and digital platforms available that allow you to track and monitor your blood sugar levels. These apps often integrate with glucose meters, CGMs, or FGM systems to collect and display your data in an organized and accessible manner. Some apps also provide additional features like meal tracking, medication reminders, and data analysis to help you better understand your blood sugar trends.

5. Paper Logs and Journals:
For those who prefer a more traditional approach, keeping a paper log or journal can be effective. Create a simple table where you can record your blood sugar readings, date, time, and any relevant notes such as meals, activities, or medication changes. This

method allows you to track your readings manually and identify patterns over time.

6. Digital Spreadsheets or Templates:
Using digital spreadsheets or templates on your computer can streamline the tracking process. Create a customized spreadsheet or use pre-existing templates to enter your blood sugar readings, date, time, and additional information as needed. Digital formats offer the advantage of easy data manipulation, graphing options, and the ability to calculate averages or trends automatically.

7. Pattern Recognition:
Beyond the specific tools mentioned above, it's important to develop the skill of pattern recognition. Look for patterns in your blood sugar readings and identify factors that contribute to fluctuations or imbalances. For example, observe how different meals, exercise routines, stress levels, medications, or sleep patterns impact your blood sugar

levels. This awareness can help you make informed choices to achieve better blood sugar control.

Remember, it's essential to follow the instructions provided with your chosen monitoring tool and consult with your healthcare provider for guidance on how frequently you should monitor your blood sugar levels. By regularly tracking and monitoring your blood sugar, you can gain valuable insights, make informed adjustments to your lifestyle, and work towards achieving optimal blood sugar regulation and overall health.

Keeping a Food and Mood Diary for Self-Awareness

Maintaining a food and mood diary can be a powerful tool for self-awareness and understanding the connection between what you eat and how you feel. By tracking your food intake and mood throughout the day, you can identify patterns, triggers, and associations that may impact your overall well-being. Here's how to effectively keep a food and mood diary:

1. Choose a Format:
Select a format that works best for you. It can be a physical journal, a digital note-taking app, or a dedicated food and mood diary app. The key is to find a method that is convenient, easy to use, and accessible at all times.

2. Record Food Intake:
Document everything you eat and drink throughout the day. Include main meals, snacks, and beverages. Be as specific as possible, noting portion sizes, ingredients, and preparation methods. Don't forget to include condiments, sauces, and any extras like sugar or cream in your coffee or tea. The more detailed your entries, the better you'll

be able to identify potential triggers or patterns.

3. Note the Time:
Record the time of each meal or snack. This helps you identify any correlations between your food intake and mood changes. It can also reveal patterns related to meal timing and how it impacts your energy levels and overall mood.

4. Rate Your Mood:
At regular intervals throughout the day, rate your mood on a scale from 1 to 10, with 1 being very low and 10 being very high. Consider factors such as happiness, energy levels, stress, anxiety, and any other emotions you may be experiencing. This helps you establish a baseline and notice any mood fluctuations in relation to your food choices.

5. Reflect on Emotional States:

Alongside your mood ratings, make notes about your emotional states, stress levels, or any significant events that occurred during the day. This can include work-related stress, personal challenges, social interactions, or any other factors that may impact your mood. Identifying emotional triggers can provide valuable insights into how your emotional well-being influences your eating habits.

6. Pay Attention to Physical Symptoms:
In addition to mood and emotions, pay attention to any physical symptoms you experience throughout the day. These can include changes in energy levels, digestive issues, headaches, bloating, or any other discomfort. Connecting physical symptoms to specific foods or situations can help you understand your body's unique responses and potential intolerances or sensitivities.

7. Be Mindful of Eating Context:

Note the circumstances surrounding your meals. Were you eating alone or with others? Did you eat in a rush or take your time to savor your food? Being mindful of the eating context helps you recognize any emotional or environmental factors that may influence your food choices and subsequent mood.

8. Review and Reflect:
Take time each day or at regular intervals to review your food and mood diary. Look for patterns, trends, or correlations between your food intake, mood, and emotional states. Ask yourself questions like: Did certain foods consistently result in a better or worse mood? Are there specific times of day when your mood tends to fluctuate? Identifying these patterns will allow you to make more informed choices about your diet and lifestyle.

9. Seek Professional Guidance:

If you notice persistent patterns or significant changes in mood that concern you, consider seeking guidance from a healthcare professional, nutritionist, or therapist. They can help you interpret the information in your food and mood diary and provide personalized recommendations based on your unique circumstances.

Remember, the goal of keeping a food and mood diary is not to judge yourself or create strict rules around eating. Instead, it is a tool for self-awareness, helping you understand how your food choices and emotional states impact each other. By cultivating this self-awareness, you can make conscious decisions to support your overall well-being and create a positive relationship with food and mood.

Chapter 8

Overcoming Challenges and Staying Motivated

Embarking on a journey to regulate your blood sugar levels and improve your health through the Glucose Goddess Method can sometimes present challenges along the way. It's important to anticipate these challenges and adopt strategies to overcome them while staying motivated and committed to your goals. Here are some helpful tips to overcome challenges and maintain your motivation:

1. Set Realistic Goals:
Set realistic and achievable goals that align with your personal circumstances. Break down your larger goals into smaller, manageable milestones. Celebrate each milestone achieved, as it will provide a sense

of accomplishment and keep you motivated to continue.

2. Educate Yourself:
Take the time to educate yourself about blood sugar regulation, nutrition, and the science behind the Glucose Goddess Method. Understanding the "why" behind your actions can empower you to make informed decisions and overcome challenges more effectively.

3. Seek Support:
Build a support system to help you navigate challenges and stay motivated. This can include family, friends, or a community of like-minded individuals who are also on a similar health journey. Share your goals and challenges with them, and lean on their encouragement and advice when needed.

4. Embrace Mindfulness and Self-Compassion:

Practice mindfulness and self-compassion throughout your journey. Be kind to yourself if you encounter setbacks or make mistakes. Treat yourself with understanding, forgiveness, and the belief that you have the capacity to learn and grow. Use mindfulness techniques to stay present, focused, and resilient during challenging times.

5. Plan Ahead:
Plan your meals, snacks, and physical activity in advance to avoid impulsive decisions or being caught unprepared. Set aside time for grocery shopping, meal prep, and scheduling workouts. By planning ahead, you can ensure you have the necessary resources and support to stick to your goals.

6. Emphasize Progress, Not Perfection:
Shift your focus from perfection to progress. Understand that setbacks or deviations from your plan are a normal part of any journey. Instead of dwelling on mistakes,

acknowledge the progress you've made and the positive changes you've experienced along the way.

7. Keep Learning and Adapting:
Stay open to learning and adapting as you progress on your journey. Continuously educate yourself about new research, strategies, and approaches to blood sugar regulation. Embrace a growth mindset, viewing challenges as opportunities for growth and improvement.

8. Celebrate Non-Scale Victories:
Recognize and celebrate non-scale victories, such as improved energy levels, better sleep, enhanced mood, or the ability to engage in activities you previously found challenging. These achievements are just as important as numerical changes on a scale and can keep you motivated during plateaus or slow progress periods.

9. Practice Self-Care:

Place an emphasis on self-care practices that are good for your body, mind, and spirit. Engage in activities you enjoy, whether it's reading a book, taking a relaxing bath, practicing yoga, or spending time in nature. Taking care of yourself holistically helps maintain motivation and reduces stress.

10. Reflect on Your Why:
Regularly reflect on the reasons why you started this journey in the first place. Connect with the deep-rooted motivations behind your desire to regulate blood sugar levels and improve your health. Revisit your goals, visualize your desired outcomes, and remind yourself of the positive impact this journey can have on your overall well-being.

Remember, challenges are a natural part of any transformative journey. By adopting these strategies and maintaining a positive mindset, you can overcome obstacles, stay motivated, and continue progressing towards optimal blood sugar control, improved health, and increased stamina through the Glucose Goddess Method.

Common Roadblocks in Blood Sugar Regulation

While striving to regulate your blood sugar levels, you may encounter certain roadblocks that can hinder your progress. Understanding and addressing these common challenges can help you navigate them more effectively. Here are some common roadblocks you may encounter in blood sugar regulation and strategies to overcome them:

1. Emotional Eating:
Emotional eating, or using food as a way to cope with emotions, can disrupt blood sugar regulation. Anxiety, depression, boredom, and stress can lead to making poor food choices or overeating. Practice mindful

eating, recognize your emotional triggers, discover healthy coping strategies like meditation or exercise, and, if necessary, get help from a therapist or counselor to stop emotional eating.

2. Unhealthy Food Cravings:
Cravings for sugary or high-carbohydrate foods can be a roadblock to maintaining stable blood sugar levels. These cravings can be caused by various factors, including imbalanced blood sugar, emotional triggers, or habitual patterns. To overcome unhealthy food cravings, focus on incorporating balanced meals with protein, healthy fats, and fiber, avoid processed foods and refined sugars, stay hydrated, and distract yourself with healthier alternatives like fresh fruit or herbal tea.

3. Lack of Meal Planning:
Failing to plan your meals in advance can lead to impulsive food choices that may disrupt blood sugar regulation. Without a

clear plan, you may be more susceptible to reaching for convenient but unhealthy options. To overcome this roadblock, dedicate time each week for meal planning, create a shopping list of nutritious ingredients, and prepare meals and snacks in advance. Having healthy options readily available will help you make better choices and maintain stable blood sugar levels.

4. Inconsistent Exercise Routine:
Regular exercise is essential for blood sugar regulation, but an inconsistent exercise routine can pose a roadblock to achieving stable levels. Lack of consistency can lead to fluctuations in insulin sensitivity and hinder the body's ability to efficiently utilize glucose. To overcome this roadblock, set realistic exercise goals, schedule workouts in advance, find activities you enjoy, and enlist a workout buddy or join a fitness community for accountability and support.

5. Sleep Deprivation:

Inadequate sleep can disrupt blood sugar regulation by affecting insulin sensitivity and increasing cravings for unhealthy foods. Lack of sleep also contributes to higher stress levels, which further impacts blood sugar balance. To overcome this roadblock, prioritize sleep hygiene by establishing a consistent sleep schedule, creating a relaxing bedtime routine, ensuring a comfortable sleep environment, and practicing stress-reducing techniques such as meditation or deep breathing exercises.

6. Medication Mismanagement: Mismanagement of diabetes medications or other medications that impact blood sugar levels can hinder your progress in blood sugar regulation. Skipping doses, taking incorrect dosages, or not adhering to prescribed treatment plans can lead to imbalances. To overcome this roadblock, work closely with your healthcare provider to understand your medication regimen, follow instructions carefully, ask questions

when in doubt, and maintain regular communication to address any concerns or adjustments needed.

7. Lack of Support and Accountability: Embarking on a blood sugar regulation journey can be challenging without a support system or accountability. It's important to surround yourself with people who understand and support your goals. Join support groups, seek guidance from healthcare professionals, or enlist the help of a health coach or registered dietitian to provide the necessary support and accountability you need.

8. Stress and Poor Stress Management: Chronic stress can significantly impact blood sugar regulation by increasing cortisol levels and affecting insulin sensitivity. Emotional eating, disturbed sleep, and irregular self-care routines can result from ineffective stress management. To overcome this roadblock, incorporate stress

management techniques such as exercise, mindfulness, meditation, deep breathing exercises, and engaging in activities you enjoy. Prioritizing self-care and seeking professional help if needed can also assist in managing stress effectively.

By recognizing and addressing these common roadblocks in blood sugar regulation, you can make adjustments to your lifestyle, develop effective strategies, and maintain stable blood sugar levels. Remember that progress takes time, and it's important to stay patient, persistent, and committed to your health goals. Consult with healthcare professionals for personalized guidance and support throughout your journey.

Strategies to Overcome Cravings and Temptations

Cravings and temptations for unhealthy foods can present significant challenges when trying to regulate your blood sugar levels. However, with the right strategies in place, you can overcome these cravings and stay on track with your goals. Here are some effective strategies to help you overcome cravings and temptations:

1. Understand the Root Cause:
Take a moment to reflect on the underlying cause of your cravings. Are they triggered by emotions, stress, boredom, or habit? Understanding the root cause can help you address the underlying issue and develop alternative coping mechanisms.

2. Distract Yourself:

When a craving hits, distract yourself by engaging in a different activity. Take a walk, call a friend, read a book, or participate in a hobby that you enjoy. Redirecting your attention away from the craving can help diminish its intensity.

3. Practice Mindful Eating:
Before giving in to a craving, pause and practice mindful eating. Pay attention to the taste, texture, and aroma of the foods you consume. Slow down, savor each bite, and listen to your body's cues of hunger and satiety. Mindful eating can help you become more aware of your body's needs and reduce impulsive eating.

4. Keep Healthy Alternatives on Hand:
Stock your pantry and refrigerator with nutritious and satisfying foods. When a craving strikes, reach for healthier alternatives that can still satisfy your taste buds. For example, choose fresh fruits, raw vegetables with hummus, or a handful of

nuts instead of sugary snacks or processed foods.

5. Stay Hydrated:
Sometimes, cravings can be a sign of dehydration. Drink a glass of water and wait a few minutes before reaching for a snack. This simple act may help alleviate the craving and provide a sense of fullness.

6. Plan Balanced Meals and Snacks:
Ensure that your meals and snacks are well-balanced, consisting of lean proteins, healthy fats, and fiber-rich carbohydrates. This combination helps stabilize blood sugar levels and keeps you feeling satisfied for longer periods, reducing the likelihood of cravings.

7. Practice Portion Control:
Rather than completely denying yourself the foods you crave, practice portion control. Allow yourself a small portion of the food you desire, savor it, and focus on enjoying

every bite. Being mindful of portion sizes can help satisfy cravings without derailing your progress.

8. Find Healthy Substitutions:
Explore healthier alternatives for your favorite indulgent foods. For example, swap sugary desserts for a fruit salad with a dollop of Greek yogurt or opt for oven-baked sweet potato fries instead of traditional fries. Finding healthier substitutes can help satisfy cravings while supporting your blood sugar regulation goals.

9. Manage Stress:
Stress can trigger cravings and temptations. Implement stress management techniques such as deep breathing exercises, meditation, yoga, or engaging in activities that help you relax and unwind. By managing stress effectively, you can reduce the likelihood of turning to unhealthy foods for comfort.

10. Seek Support and Accountability:
Reach out to a support system of family, friends, or a community that shares similar health goals. Share your struggles and victories with them, and seek their support and encouragement when cravings and temptations arise. Having accountability and encouragement from others can be instrumental in overcoming challenges.

11. Celebrate Non-Food Rewards:
Reward yourself for progress and achievements with non-food rewards. Treat yourself to a massage, buy yourself a new book, or engage in an activity you love. Non-food rewards help reinforce positive behaviors and motivate you to stay on track.

Remember, overcoming cravings and temptations requires practice and patience. Be kind to yourself and embrace the journey towards balanced and healthy eating. With time and consistent effort, you can develop healthier habits and maintain stable blood sugar levels.

Building a Support Network for Continued Success

When it comes to regulating your blood sugar levels and maintaining a healthy lifestyle, having a strong support network can make a significant difference in your success. Building a support network provides you with encouragement, accountability, and resources to overcome challenges and stay motivated. Here are some strategies to help you build a support network for continued success:

1. Share Your Goals:
Openly communicate your health goals with your family, friends, and loved ones. Let them know why blood sugar regulation is important to you and how it contributes to

your overall well-being. Sharing your goals creates a support system that can provide motivation and understanding throughout your journey.

2. Join Support Groups:
Look for local or online support groups focused on blood sugar regulation, diabetes management, or general health and wellness. These groups provide a space for sharing experiences, exchanging tips and advice, and finding inspiration from others who are on a similar path. Participating in discussions and engaging with the community can give you a sense of belonging and support.

3. Seek Professional Guidance:
Consult with healthcare professionals who specialize in diabetes management, nutrition, or blood sugar regulation. They can provide expert advice, personalized guidance, and ongoing support. Regular check-ins with your healthcare team can

help you stay on track, make necessary adjustments to your plan, and address any concerns or questions you may have.

4. Enlist a Workout Buddy:
Find a workout buddy who shares similar health goals. Exercising with a partner can make workouts more enjoyable, provide accountability, and increase motivation. Whether it's a friend, family member, or colleague, having someone to share your fitness journey with can make a significant difference in staying consistent and reaching your exercise goals.

5. Connect Online:
Utilize online platforms and social media to connect with individuals who are also focused on blood sugar regulation and overall health. Join online communities, follow health and wellness influencers, and engage in conversations related to your goals. Online platforms can provide a wealth

of information, support, and inspiration from people all around the world.

6. Involve Your Loved Ones:
Engage your loved ones in your health journey. Encourage them to participate in activities such as meal planning, cooking nutritious meals together, or joining you in physical activities. Involving your loved ones not only strengthens your support network but also creates a healthier environment for everyone involved.

7. Consider a Health Coach or Mentor:
Hiring a health coach or finding a mentor who specializes in blood sugar regulation and health can provide you with personalized guidance, accountability, and support. They can help you develop strategies, overcome obstacles, and navigate through the complexities of maintaining healthy blood sugar levels.

8. Attend Workshops or Classes:

Look for workshops, classes, or educational programs in your community that focus on nutrition, cooking, fitness, or blood sugar regulation. These events provide opportunities to learn from experts, connect with like-minded individuals, and expand your knowledge and skills related to maintaining a healthy lifestyle.

9. Celebrate Achievements Together:
Share your successes and milestones with your support network. Celebrate achievements, whether they are small or significant, and acknowledge the hard work and dedication that led to those accomplishments. Positive reinforcement from your support network can boost your motivation and reinforce your commitment to your health goals.

10. Be Supportive of Others:
Support is a two-way street. Be there for others who are also on a health journey, whether they are friends, family members,

or fellow community members. Offer encouragement, listen actively, and share your experiences and knowledge when appropriate. By being supportive of others, you create a reciprocal and uplifting environment.

Building a support network takes time and effort, but the benefits are invaluable. Surrounding yourself with individuals who understand your journey, provide encouragement, and offer practical support can greatly enhance your chances of long-term success in blood sugar regulation and overall health. Together, you can overcome challenges, celebrate victories, and create a positive and sustainable lifestyle.

Conclusion

Congratulations on completing "The Glucose Goddess Method: A Comprehensive Guide to Regulate Your Blood Sugar Levels, Transform Your Health, and Regain Stamina." Throughout this book, we have explored the intricacies of blood sugar regulation, the science behind it, and effective strategies for achieving and maintaining stable blood sugar levels.

By understanding the importance of blood sugar regulation and its impact on your overall health, you have gained valuable insights into the role of insulin, glycemic index, and the various factors that can influence your blood sugar levels. Through assessments, diagnostic tests, and self-awareness, you have learned how to monitor your blood sugar levels and identify signs of imbalance.

The Glucose Goddess Method has provided you with a holistic approach to blood sugar balance, encompassing the four pillars of nutrition, exercise, stress management, and sleep. You have discovered the power of nourishing your body with wholesome foods, implementing portion control, and incorporating superfoods and supplements for optimal blood sugar support.

Furthermore, you have learned how physical activity and tailored workout routines can play a pivotal role in regulating blood sugar levels, boosting stamina, and improving overall health. Stress management techniques and relaxation practices have been explored to help you address the connection between stress and blood sugar.

Through tracking your progress, using diagnostic tools, and keeping a food and mood diary, you have developed a deeper understanding of your body's responses and the impact of your lifestyle choices.

Moreover, you have explored common roadblocks, strategies to overcome cravings and temptations, and the importance of building a strong support network.

Remember, blood sugar regulation is a journey that requires commitment, patience, and self-care. Embrace the principles and philosophy of The Glucose Goddess Method, and continue implementing the strategies and tools you have acquired. Be kind to yourself and celebrate your progress, no matter how small, as each step forward brings you closer to optimal health and vitality.

Always consult with healthcare professionals for personalized advice, and adapt the strategies to suit your individual needs. With dedication and perseverance, you have the power to transform your health, regulate your blood sugar levels, and reclaim your stamina.

Here's to a vibrant and balanced life filled with energy, wellness, and the joys of optimal blood sugar control. May you continue to thrive on your journey to becoming the Glucose Goddess.

Wishing you health and happiness,

Margaret R. Harris

Printed in Great Britain
by Amazon

24871098R00096